# DEDICATION

This is dedicated to my family. It is also dedicated to those who are seeking the healthier lifestyle which starts with the right diet.

I had issues finding the right diet and I gained a lot of excess weight as a result of it. Thankfully I am now on track with the help of my family.

# TABLE OF CONTENTS

# Paleo Diet Plan: The Simple Guide for Paleo for Beginners

**The Right Diet with the Paleo Diet Plan**

By: Andryan Coombs

9781632874672

# PUBLISHERS NOTES

### Disclaimer – Speedy Publishing, LLC

This publication is intended to provide helpful and informative material. It is not intended to diagnose, treat, cure, or prevent any health problem or condition, nor is intended to replace the advice of a physician. No action should be taken solely on the contents of this book. Always consult your physician or qualified health-care professional on any matters regarding your health and before adopting any suggestions in this book or drawing inferences from it.

The author and publisher specifically disclaim all responsibility for any liability, loss or risk, personal or otherwise, which is incurred as a consequence, directly or indirectly, from the use or application of any contents of this book.

Any and all product names referenced within this book are the trademarks of their respective owners. None of these owners have sponsored, authorized, endorsed, or approved this book.

Always read all information provided by the manufacturers' product labels before using their products. The author and publisher are not responsible for claims made by manufacturers.

***This book was originally printed before 2014. This is an adapted reprint by Speedy Publishing, LLC with newly updated content designed to help readers with much more accurate and timely information and data.***

Speedy Publishing, LLC

40 E Main Street,

Newark

Delaware

19711

Contact Us: 1-888-248-4521

Website: http://www.speedypublishing.com

REPRINTED Paperback Edition: ISBN: 9781632874672

Manufactured in the United States of America

# INTRODUCTION

Anyone who takes a sustained look at the obesity numbers in the present global population will notice that they are rising fast. Despite the advancement in technology, healthcare and education, people are still making mistakes in how they eat. The current state of obesity in the world in 2013 calls for a return to the Paleo diet, the right way to cope with evolution. The present obesity debacle arises from the fact that people are taking up a lifestyle that is not optimal for their existence on earth and these behaviors leave the body with too many extra calories than it requires.

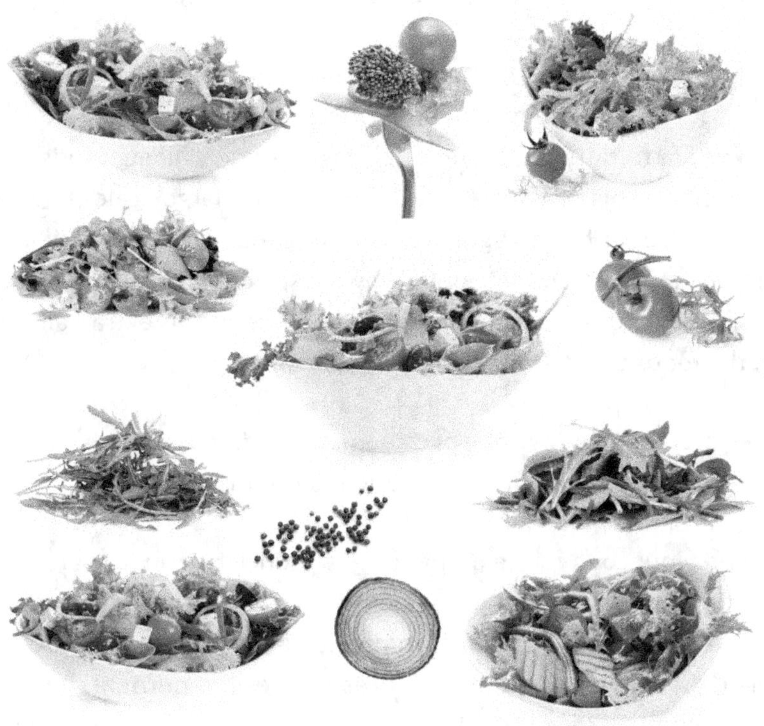

*Paleo Diet Plan*

The Paleo diet derives its philosophy from the fact that people who inhabited the earth more than 10,000 years ago did not eat any processed food yet they were healthy and not obese. They did not experience modern-day diseases like arthritis, cardiovascular complications and cancers. So based on this fact, anyone wishing to enjoy a healthy Paleo diet and regain their health should simply ask themselves whether a caveman would eat what the person is about to eat. If the answer is yes, then it is a go-ahead for eating that particular food but if it's no, then it would be a hint to stop taking the kind of food.

In 2005, the Paleo diet went mainstream after famous people started asking their followers to embrace it. Since then various authoritative materials such as books and articles have been published to explain its benefits to health and fitness.

In the past, human bodies were wired to cushion themselves against any form of food scarcity. That was the beginning of the attraction to fatty foods and other high calorie yielding foods. The present problem is that, technology and large-scale farming brought about by the agrarian revolution has made it possible to create excess food. People nowadays eat because it feels convenient to eat and not because they need the extra calories, in the foods that they take.

The problem with most of the modern diet is that it lacks a balanced supply of both macro and micronutrients.

When your body is experiencing a deficiency in a particular nutrient, it will initiate a hunger stimulus in your brain that will cause you to eat more. Unfortunately, if you do not go on to eat the right kind of food that produces the desired nutrient, you will end up with excess and still lack what you need. Thus it is a major cause of obesity.

Now many modern fitness diet advocates call for a calorie limitation as a weight loss measure. This is beneficial only to a point. Remember that, without the right supply of all micro nutrients, your body will still cause hunger stimulus that causes you to break your fitness diet and eat in excess.

You can succeed at a health fitness diet without the urges to binge eat by taking up the Paleo diet. It includes unprocessed meats, fresh fruits and vegetables as well as nuts. This combination has a lot of fiber that leaves you filled without giving you excess calories. The Paleo diet is low on refined sugars and oils. The elimination of these two main ingredients that lead to obesity creates a calorie deficit and a nutrient surplus that leads to successful weight loss. Indeed, the time to take up the Paleo diet is now. Journey with us as we embark on living life the Paleo way

# CHAPTER 1- WHAT IS THE PALEO DIET?

Currently a lot of people are talking about the Paleo diet; some people also refer to it as the caveman diet. Well this may be true due to the fact that it originated from our ancient ancestors.

Humans have changed drastically in times of technology, culture and diet. On this particular discussion, our interest is on diet. After the Neolithic period, humans started practicing agriculture hence a variety of ingredients become available for consumption changing our diet immensely.

Paleo eaters argue that as much as our environment has changed, our bodies have not had any change compared to our ancestors with our genes having changed by a mere 0.001% therefore our diets should not change as well. Modern foods have been associated with a lot of medical conditions such as cancer due to the ingredients they contain while they may be tasty and appealing, natural foods are healthier.

This brings us to the popular question, what exactly is the Paleo diet?

This is a low sugar; high protein and low sodium diet that is meant to provide optimum health by following in our ancestors footsteps that lived in the Paleolithic age. The basic principle about this diet is optimum health but is also a good alternative if your aim is to lose weight.

A lot of evidence has been found to prove that our ancestors had the finest health and this is attributed to their diet. Different people may have various definitions to answer this question but there are similarities in all these definitions i.e. minimally processed, locally available, in-season foods. A good way to also define this diet is by saying what it is not i.e. Paleo diet is not any industrial refined oil, sugar, dairy, alcohol etc.

Pastured, free-range chicken, grass-fed beef and anything organic are the most preferred foods for a Paleo dieter. In terms of proteins, seafood/fish, poultry, lean meats, wild game are favored because they contain less saturated fats unlike processed meats.

When it comes to nuts or seeds, the ones with the most concentration of omega-3 i.e. walnuts, macadamia, almonds and cashews are the best. Fruits with low glycemic index e.g. tomatoes, melons, onions and broccoli are favored unlike modern fruits to be large and look good. Herbs and spices are recommended regardless of whether they have been processes since they are organic anyways i.e. vinegar.

Fast foods or foods in flashy wrappers are attractive, sweet and tempting; I bet you always salivate when you walk past a fast food café. The smell of fries, burgers and a drink of cold soda, well it is completely normal to feel that way (almost everyone feels that) but after trying Paleo for about 6 months, you would be surprised that a diet soda tastes very different than what you used to know, you can literally taste all the chemicals in it.

The Paleo diet is growing daily as more people are getting concerned with what they eat, we are looking for ways to prevent or lose weight. By recreating our early human diet, we are getting in touch with the ancient taste while reaping all the benefits that come with it. I believe this has answered the question, what exactly is the Paleo diet and a couple of the foods recommended.

# CHAPTER 2- THE REVIVAL OF THE PALEO DIET

As we have discussed, the Paleo diet is based on ancient diet of man which included animals and wild plants that were consumed 2. 5 million years ago during the Paleolithic era.

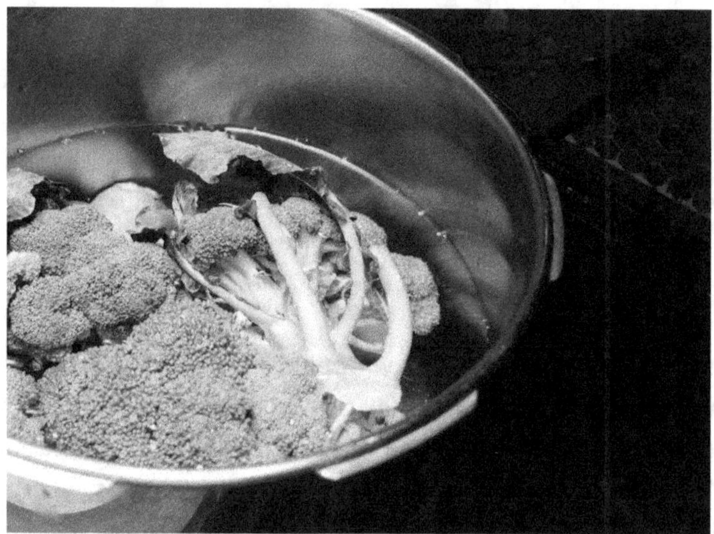

It is preservative and gluten free. It is commonly centered on foods like eggs, fish, grass fed pasture raised meats, vegetables, potatoes, roots, fungi, fruits, nuts, potatoes, dairy products, grains, refined salt, refined sugar, legumes and processed oils. But let's now retrace the steps and cover how this diet came back from extinction and learn the history of it

The history of the Paleo diet can be traced back to 1975 when Walter L. Voegtlin a gastroenterologist published a book that highlighted the modern version of the diet. He arrived at his revelations after studying eating habits of the Paleolithic age while looking for a cure for Crohn's disease, colitis and irritable bowel syndrome. Diet from early man seemed to have adverse effects on the conditions where patients improved quickly without any side effects.

His version on the diet was based on the fact that there has not been much human genetic change since the Paleolithic era. He was more interested in the carnivorous history of man. He confirmed that humans are supposed to primarily feed on fats, proteins with little carbohydrates.

A decade later Professor Melvin Konner an anthropologist took the concepts to the scientific community with the assistance of an associate called Boyd Eaton. They did this by publishing a paper on the concepts in the New England Journal of Medicine. Professionals in the medical field started discussing the diet which is a very important stage of the history of the Paleo diet. A high percentage was convinced about the advantages of the diet.

Three years down the line Eaton, Konner and Marjorie Shostak published a book on the diet. The book was however written with a twist. Instead of focusing on the foods that should not be included in the diet, they talked about the importance of eating same portion of carbohydrates, fats and proteins similar to the Paleolithic era diet.

Their version had some foods that were not allowed by Voegtlin. Their diet allowed permitted agricultural foods like whole grain bread, brown rice, potatoes and dairy products like skimmed milk that were not featured on the original diet. They work on the rationale that the nutrient proportion and not food choice was what made the Paleolithic diet healthy.

Momentum for the diet continued to grow even in the 1990s as more nutritionists and medical professionals began to back the theory. More doctors started recommending it to their patients as part of a healthy eating plan for the sick patients and even the ones who were well. Most of them relied on the original concept where the diet consisted of the foods present before the introduction of agriculture.

As the years went by more people were drawn to the diet. Although it was hotly debated, it was still accepted in various circles. Today there are very many books and websites written on the diet as more and more people embrace it. At this point, it does not show any signs of dying away.

# CHAPTER 3- IS IT WORTH IT?

The Paleo diet has become more popular due to all of the health benefits of it. If you are thinking about going on this diet yourself, there are a lot of reasons to seriously consider it. This can become a way of life that can make you healthy and really change your outlook on food!

**Benefits of Going Paleo**

**Weight Loss**

Losing weight is hard for most people because they are either going on crazy diets or they are simply eating foods that aren't good for them. The Paleo diet can help you lose weight because the foods you will be eating are healthy and good for you! These can help you cut out fats and calories that you just don't need. This will result in weight loss that doesn't come from you starving or having to give up eating foods you enjoy. Most people continuously lose weight while on this diet because it's so healthy and easy to stick with.

**Energy**

Have you ever felt really tired and lethargic after eating a big meal full of carbohydrates and fats? Fast foods and unhealthy meals can make you feel terrible because they don't have anything good for you inside of them. By changing the foods you eat to those that are healthy, you will have more energy overall and feel great each day!

Getting the proper vitamins and nutrients in your diet can make a huge difference with the way you feel and really help you get extra energy you have been lacking.

*Paleo Diet Plan*
**Nutrition**

When eating a diet of junk food, candy, sugar, carbs and other bad foods it's difficult to get the proper vitamins and nutrients that are essential for a healthy body. When you switch to the Paleo way of life you will easily be able to get the nutrients that you need. All of the foods you eat will be packed full of things like fiber, vitamin a, vitamin c and other nutrients that are great for your body. When you have better nutrition in your life you will feel better and look better!

**Allergies**

The junk foods that people eat today are packed full of toxic ingredients that can easily hurt the body. For example, gluten intolerance is one of the biggest problems most people have today. The Paleo diet will make it possible to eat good food without having to worry about food allergens. Of course you should pay attention to what you eat if you are sensitive to certain things, but you won't have to deal with any chemicals or hidden toxins.

**Recipes**

There are a lot of different recipes you can make for the Paleo diet. These are easy to find and they taste great as well. These can help you find new foods that you enjoy eating and that are really good for you. When you aren't starving yourself or feeling deprived it will be easy to eat healthy and change the way you eat on a daily basis.

All of these benefits are worth considering if you want to change your eating habits and your health. The Paleo way of life is easy to adopt and can make you feel great from day one.

# CHAPTER 4- THE PALEO DIET COMPARED TO OTHER DIETS

Paleolithic diet, also called as Stone Age diet, ancient man diet or caveman's diet, is a result of extensive work of gastroenterologist Walter L. Voegtlin. It was found that modern humans have evolved a genetic capacity for the diet of prehistoric humans but not for the agriculture diet. This is the main reason for the deluge of health issues that mankind faces today.

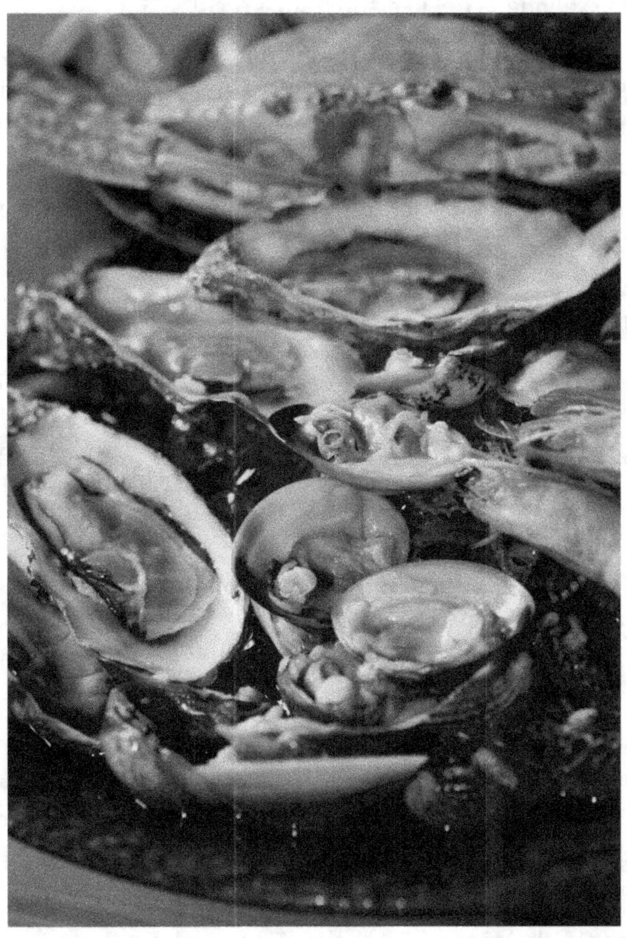

*Paleo Diet Plan*

Paleo diets are centered on recipes mainly consisting fish, grass-fed pasture raised meats, vegetables, fruit, roots, and nuts. Foods cultivated through extensive agriculture practices like grains and legumes are avoided. Dairy products, salt, refined sugar, and processed foods are also not consumed.

Paleo diets are mainly consumed for their nutritional content. The ability of Paleo diets to help maintain weight despite their high nutritional value can be attributed to two kinds of fiber components in them - The soluble and insoluble fiber. Soluble fiber in Paleo diet, called beta glucans, can be dissolved in water and on dissolving, a gel like substance results.

This can trap bad cholesterol particles i.e. LDL. This action helps prevent the onset of heart diseases occurring due to the accumulation of fat in the blood vessels, mainly arteries. Many scientific studies have found that even moderate consumption of Paleo foods can help reduce cholesterol accumulation by 3%. In the process of combating LDL from the food consumed, the good cholesterol (HDL) is not affected.

The gelatinous substance tends to the change the properties of the digested food in the stomach. Due to this change, the contents tend to move slowly, thereby giving a feeling of fullness and reduction in unnecessary excessive intake of food. The prolonged stay also results in complete digestion activity by the enzymes present in the stomach and intestines. The contents are changed to the extent that they slow down but not completely stop.

Another function of soluble fiber and the resultant gel is regulation of excess nutrients in blood. Since soluble fiber prolongs digestion, there is time for nutrients to enter the blood stream without having the body intake more. This function is very important in the case of Diabetics. Since carbohydrates and sugar molecules undergo slow digestion due to soluble fiber, the body has ample time to convert these into energy before the requirement to eat arises again. Hence pile up of sugar in blood is reduced.

The Insoluble fiber serves to push the contents in the intestines. This it does by absorbing water and becoming heavy. The excess weight and expansion exerts more pressure in the Gastrointestinal (GI) tract and pushes the contents out of the body smoothly. Hence regulated bowel movement is achieved and constipation prevented.

Paleo diets help maintain pH balance in the intestines. pH is an indicator of acidity. If the contents of the stomach are acidic and the condition turns chronic then chances of colorectal cancer increases many fold. Paleo diet serves to negate this effect of pH change. They also contain Lignans which have been found to reduce risks of hormonal cancers. Several researchers have found a relation between decreased risks, due to Paleo diet consumption, of breast cancer in women. These women had lower levels of estrogen which reduced the risk.

The natural carbohydrate content in Paleo diets are a rich source of energy. This energy is released instantly and it has been proven that they can enhance work performance in individuals within 30-40 minutes after consumption. This is ideal when you wake up in the morning and don't fell like having a lot but want to consume just enough to keep you going till lunch.

There are many other benefits of Paleo diets. Essential fatty acids present have been found to keep a check on the blood pressure. They are also known to help with circulatory problems. The amino acids present are essential for protein creation which are an important source of energy for the body. Many minerals present in Paleo diets help in improving the oxygen carrying capacity of blood. The most prominent are Iron and magnesium. These are present in adequate quantities. Regular intake of Paleo diets can help keep in check the blood pressure. Consumption of Paleo diets results in general well being. They are easily available, inexpensive and can be part of your full day program.

Paleo Diet is also noted for its no milk stand. One may why milk and dairy products are not included. Milk and dairy products are major causes of health related issues like cardiovascular disease. As most of them are processed, the naturalness in them lost and hence is avoided in Paleo diet.

**Why No Milk?**

Milk allergy is an immune system reaction when milk is consumed. Proteins present in milk are the cause of the allergy. Some people have an immune system that simple can't adapt to these proteins and consider the proteins as foreign bodies.

Hence the immune system rushes to counter and flush these proteins out of the body. It is like any other food allergic reaction. Milk allergy should not be confused with lactose intolerance or Milk protein intolerance. Milk allergy is purely an immune system reaction while lactose intolerance is the inability of the produce to the enzyme Lactase to digest lactose present in milk. Milk protein intolerance is a delayed reaction to a food protein. It is not an allergy reaction and cannot be detected by allergy test though the symptoms are similar to milk allergy. Usually milk allergy is seen in infants and children and lactose intolerance on consumption of large quantities of milk.

Allergy reaction to milk is caused by mainly two proteins- casein and whey. Casein is the largest component of milk (the curd part of milk) and is the main cause for allergy. The remaining part of milk i.e. the watery part is whey. Infants and children are likely to be allergic to milk. Very rarely do adults develop it if they dint have it as children. However most of them tend to get rid of it by the time they turn 10. But some a good number of them also fail to leave it behind and tend to suffer when they are adults. A study also found that the symptoms are not fixed. Over a period of time, the allergy can manifest itself in a not encountered previously in the sufferer.

The best way to avoid an allergy is avoiding milk and milk products. Though there is medication, milk avoidance is a sure shot.

If you want to lose weight, then there are several options. So how do you know which of those work and which of those don't? Well simply going by the number of people using the program is testimonial enough of how good a program. Paleo diet is one such program that is tried and tested by several people who wanted to lose weight and wanted to get in shape in little time. It is a healthy diet but not a crash diet. There is no need to starve or go on a diet that is binding. There are several options but modern processed foods are a NO because they were not available to our ancestors. With Paleo diet you can stay healthy, build strength and lose weight but not muscle mass. You become leaner and fitter, without hurting your metabolism.

Research suggests that when you go on a restricted diet for a week, the body is just about to enter the starvation mode. At this point you cheat by indulging in your favorite food. This way you keep it from entering starvation as the metabolism is not shut down and continues to burn fat. Unlike diet programs Paleo diet works with the body and not against it.

The Paleo diet program is essentially about what food needs to be eaten and what should not be eaten. There is a schedule which you have to follow in order to benefit the most. There is no idea of cheating in this diet program as it suggests lifestyle changes while cheating implies you can retain some of your older eating habits. This helps you get rid of weight but also satisfy your food cravings.

When you are on Paleo diet you are losing weight permanently. Unlike dieting programs, you won't put on weight once you lose it. You are not going to harm your metabolism or lose any muscle mass. You don't have to count calories worriedly when you are on Paleo diet nor will you need to punish yourself because Paleo recipes are delicious.

It does not matter if obesity is in your genes as Paleo diet can help combat this factor. Several extremely overweight people have been able to drastically lose weight and reclaim their lives.

Omega 3 fatty acids in Paleo diets have been shown to prevent cancer and reduce tumor growth in those with cancers. The immune system has a better chance to fight off cancer because it is strengthened. A study conducted on patients who were to undergo surgery for tumor removal showed that on consumption of Paleo diets their tumor growth had slowed down considerably. LDL content is the body is also significantly decreased in the body without harming HDL.

This reduces the risk of formation of plaques in arteries thereby reducing the chances of heart attacks. They have also been shown to help keep the blood pressure in check.

The benefits of Paleo diet can be seen in as little as two weeks within which the body starts the detox process. These first few days might prove tough as you have to go on a restricted diet of high nutrition fruits and vegetables, lean meat and eggs. Eating healthy is the key to the success of the program. Paleo diet fat loss programs detail healthy food recipes that are not only easy to make, but are delicious enough to replace junk food. You can also learn how you can control frequent snacking and your food cravings.

Paleo diet also does not allow you to indulge in alcohol. The effects of alcohol are well known and many research studies have weighed various effects it has on the body.

They had all concluded that alcohol is bad when taken in excess and the required quantity has to been taken only to provide warmth to the body in areas of extremely low temperature. Alcohol is an intoxicant and any amount of consumption will get the body working to get rid of it. Excessive intake will cause violent reactions. A person will lose muscle control and strength. It also affects the tongue and results in slurred speech.

Alcohol affects sense of orientation. The balance mechanism is present in the inner ear and its consumption results in changes of fluid pressure in the ear. Alcohol also affects the nervous system causing a sense of euphoria which can result in accidents and drunken behavior. Alcohol is dangerous for pregnant mothers. Consumption can result in babies born with mental and physical disabilities. Since alcohol runs in the blood stream the babies would also be infused with it and can cause irregularities in their delicate systems.

Chronic consumption of alcohol results in the damage of liver. Alcohol can cause liver inflammation and corrosion. Cirrhosis is a disease of the liver where liver cells are damaged and the body needs a liver transplant as the existing liver has lost its regenerative capacity. Liver is the most affected organ as its function is to metabolize alcohol.

Heart disease is another major ill effect. It causes the weakening of heart muscle and thereby increases the chance of a stroke or arrest. Since it tends to elevate blood pressure, alcohol pushes the heart to work harder and over time results in heart failure. Due to the increased pressure, the vessel walls also get damaged. Pancreas is also affected. The organ helps in production of enzymes necessary for digestion.

Excess long term drinking can cause swelling of pancreas. The condition is called Pancreatis. The pancreas is also responsible for insulin regulation and if they are affected by alcohol, diabetes can result.

Kidneys which are filters of the body can take a beating due to excessive alcohol consumption. Once the kidneys are damaged, the body accumulates toxins. Alcohol usage in modern times is also associated with depression and insomnia. People who consume it have fitful and erratic sleep patterns.

Vitamin A is an anti-oxidant, helping prevent cells from the harmful effects of oxygen. Oxygen, despite its essentiality for living life can also be damaging. Paleo Diet is rich in anti oxidants and along with other vitamins, it neutralizes free radicals that can radicalize healthy cells and damage them. It was also observed that prolonged use of Diet tend to reduce carcinogenic risk and other DNA mutations. The presence of anti oxidants can make the skin remain healthy and blemish free. They can reduce the ageing of skin and lend it a young feel and also helps prevent night blindness. The vitamin A in Diet is responsible for this. Other benefits of the Diet due are strengthening of bones, prevents heart diseases and help combat respiratory problems like asthma.

Paleo Diet can improve clotting properties of blood in those with problems like hemophilia. Women with excessive menstrual bleeding can also benefit from the diet because it is holistic in terms of nutrition. Many women have reported that such a diet helps in normalizing menstrual cycles and helps make the bleeding normal. People suffering with osteoporosis, mainly women in the menopause phase can also greatly benefit from it. Their bones are strengthened and they have fewer fractures just like our ancestors.

These foods also offer protection of the body from sun burns. The vitamin E present prevents the skin from the damage that ultra violet rays of the sun can cause. Diet also protects the body against skin diseases like psoriasis and skin allergic inflammation.

Vitamin C present in the foods is another anti oxidant. It helps in maintaining the structure and elasticity of blood vessels. Blood vessels have to be in proper shape for the blood to flow with the right pressure and to prevent undue stress on the heart. Vitamin C also helps in maintaining the heart muscle itself.

Magnesium, potassium and calcium are present in high concentrations in Paleo Diets. These three minerals help the body regulate blood flow and control pressure in small capillaries. When people with high blood pressure started consuming Paleo foods, over a period of a week their blood pressure fluctuations decreased by about 30 percent.

The Phytochemical sulphorane helps prevent gene modification by diseases like cancer. It also helps the body fight cancer and prevents it. Sulphorane is also beneficial for liver. It was shown that liver with injury recuperated faster on consuming Paleo foods.

As was mentioned earlier Paleo Diet is also known for its fiber content. The ability of Paleo foods to help maintain weight despite its high nutritional value can be attributed to the fiber in it. Fiber can be dissolved in water and on dissolving a gel like substance results. This can trap bad cholesterol particles i.e. LDL. This action helps prevent the onset of heart diseases occurring due to the accumulation of fat in blood vessels, mainly arteries. In the process of combating LDL from the food consumed, the good cholesterol (HDL) is not affected.

# CHAPTER 5- GETTING READY FOR THE PALEO DIET

The Paleo diet is quite simple to follow since it doesn't involve counting calories or other restrictions. It focuses on eating natural and fresh foods just like the hunters and gatherers did. As long as you are eating fresh sea food, lean meat, nuts, fruits and vegetables as provided in this diet then you can take as much as you wish without counting carbohydrates, fats and calories.

Before you embark on the Paleo diet you must have an inquiring and open mind. You have to sit down and decide when to start and what to eat in the first week. Primarily, if you choose to begin with a full on diet then you will experience an adjustment period. This period will most likely involve some mental, emotional and physical withdrawal symptoms as you begin changing your usual eating habits.

Because of the adjustment phase, it is advisable to start the diet when your life is relatively calm and without stressful situations. Some people can experience a slight headache while others show symptoms of flu for just a few days. The adjustment period can last for a week or two. During this phase, there is a feeling of fatigue, dizziness and a powerful craving for some delicious carbohydrate foods.

**How to Manage Cravings and Symptoms**

One most strange aspect of human psychology is that people crave foods that have no nutritional value for their bodies. This is exactly true for dairy products and grains; therefore people who start the Paleo diet experience an intense craving for such foods.

*Paleo Diet Plan*

Here are some things to do to make the change of lifestyle a bit easier.

**Drink a Lot of Water**

Include garlic and onions in your food. They are rich in sulphur and amino acids. Sulphur is an important component of the detox system.

Add plenty of turmeric in your food. Turmeric is a strong anti - inflammatory and antioxidant agent.

Cook your meals with coconut oil or olive oil. Oily fish is also very good.

**Planning Your Paleo Diet**

You must not embark on the diet before planning what foods you are going to take during the first week. Buy the things that are needed in advance to avoid reaching out for some sugary snacks immediately craving starts. It is wise to have adequate supply of snacks like walnuts, almonds, peanuts and fruits. When planning your Paleo diet you have to focus on mealtimes. Here is a sample meal plan.

**Breakfast**

-Eggs, mushroom, garlic, onions and steamed spinach

-Use coconut oil

-Avocado Lunch

-Chicken salad with red onions

-Herb, olive oil and lemon juice dressing

-Pecans, cantaloupe and blackberries Snack

- ¼ cup macadamias Dinner

-Venison steak

-Ginger cabbage and olive oil

-Steamed summer squash with lemon juice, cinnamon and coconut milk

**Desert**

-Shaved almonds

Your first shopping trip ought to include fresh vegetables, lean meat, chicken, fish and some allowed snacks. Buy load of herbs, coconut oil, Epsom salt, olive oil and anything that will help you survive the adjustment phase.

**Taking Care of Yourself**

It is a great idea to observe your body's reaction to the new diet. There are plenty of nutrients and no filers in the Paleo diet. Many people experience a detoxification period where their bodies learn how to use fats as the main source of energy instead of carbohydrates.

# CHAPTER 6- WHAT TO EAT AND WHAT TO AVOID

If you would like to adopt the Paleo diet, here is the chapter for you that enumerates what to eat and what to avoid while on the diet plan. Read on.

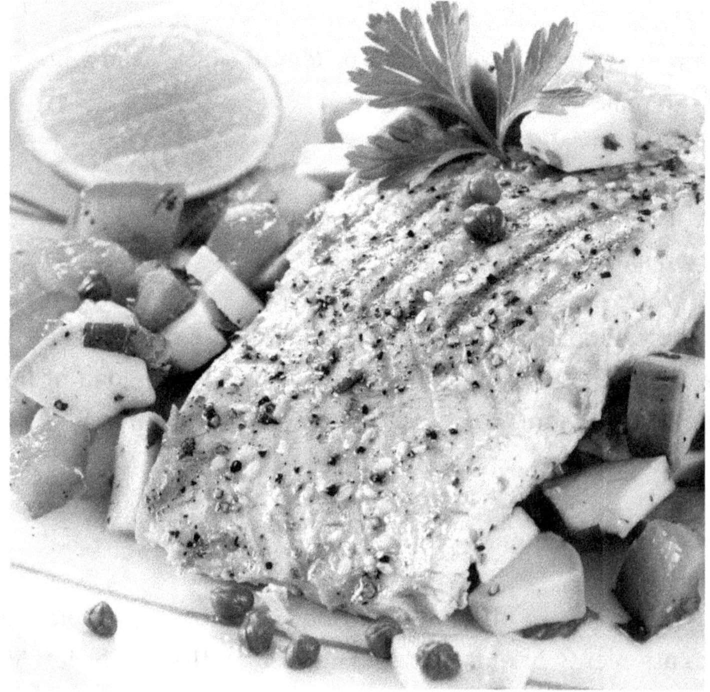

**What to Eat**

**Vegetables**

Vegetables are highly encouraged. However, the consumption of starchy vegetables such as yams, sweet potatoes, potatoes and cassava should be limited or better avoided. Propagators of the

Paleo diet are of the opinion that any vegetable that cannot be consumed raw should be eliminated from the diet.

## Fruits

Fruits such as berries, apples and oranges are perfectly fine for the diet but you should consume them in moderation. Equally important, don't consume fruits in their dried version e.g. dried apricots or their dried products. Again, fruits such as grapes and bananas should be avoided as they contain a lot of sugar.

## Eggs and Meat

The Paleo diet advocates for the consumption of meat and eggs. However, you should stick to the grass-fed products and avoid meats that contain additives and preservatives in the meat you consume. Pork, game, beef, chicken, turkey and fish are the best for this diet. Chicken eggs, quail eggs and any other type of eggs are included in the diet.

## Seeds and Nuts

All nuts and seeds, save for peanuts, are allowed. Peanuts are exempted because they are legumes. However, if you'd like to lose weight, you should moderate your consumption to about four ounces every day. Coconut and almond flour are also included in this list.

## Oils

Unprocessed oils such as coconut oil, walnut oil, tallow, lard, olive oil and canola oil are highly recommended. Fish oil supplements are also encouraged. However, processed vegetable and hydrogenated oils are heavily discouraged. Furthermore, the existence of processed oils came with agriculture and industrialization.

## Beverages

Drinking a lot of water is highly emphasized in the Paleo diet. Plain tea "without milk" as well as fruit and vegetable juices are also allowed.

## Foods to Avoid

### Grains

The entire family of cereal grains should be avoided. This includes wheat, rice, corn, oats and barley. Proponents of the diet put much emphasis on avoiding white flour and rice as they contain refined carbohydrates.

### Legumes

As aforementioned, legumes are not included in the Paleo diet plan. This includes all kinds of beans; string beans, kidney beans, black beans, soybeans, lima beans and mung beans. Again, black-eye peas, sugar-snap peas, snow peas and peanuts should be avoided.

### Dairy Products

Dairy products such as butter, yogurt, skim milk, whole milk, cream, cheese, ice cream and dairy creamer are prohibited.

You should also steer away from alcohol, soft drinks, refined sweeteners and iodized salt. Processed foods should also be eliminated from the diet. It's important to note that the Paleolithic diet offers a number of benefits including weight loss, increase activity and general body health. Adopt it, stick to it and you'll gradually start to enjoy its benefits.

# CHAPTER 7- A DAY IN THE LIFE OF A PALEO DIET

On any given day a Paleo meal plan may include foods like vegetables, eggs, fresh fruits, nuts, lean meats and seafood. Such a meal provides you with nutrients such as phyto-nutrients, soluble fiber, antioxidants, carbohydrates and monounsaturated fats.

When preparing a Paleo meal, you need to focus on poultry, red meat, fish, eggs, nuts and seeds, vegetables and fruits. A small amount of honey, plant oils and dried fruits can also be included in your meals. Avoid any processed food with artificial ingredients, refined sugars, grains, salt and saturated fats.

Once you have made an effort to reduce your intake of packaged foods and grains, then you are ready to start following a daily Paleo diet. Read on to see a sample daily meal plan on the Paleo diet.

**Paleo Breakfast**

Eating simply is one of the basics of the Paleo diet; simply generally means that you eat less food. For your breakfast you can prepare two scrambled eggs and turkey bacon. This a good and hearty meal that can be combined with Paleo pancakes. You can prepare a Paleo pancake by combining one cup of almond flour, three eggs, ¼ teaspoon of a vanilla extract and ¼ teaspoon of cinnamon. This will give you around 4 to 5 pancakes.

You can also try spinach and tomato omelet together with strawberries.

*Andryan Coombs*
**Paleo Lunch**

You can try a protein-style hamburgers or a big salad. Begin with a combination of greens, sliced carrots, sliced avocado, diced red pepper, raw mushrooms sliced, chopped walnuts, diced spring onions, lemon juice and equal amounts of olive oil.

**Paleo Dinner**

Prepare any combination of eggs, vegetables and meat. A sofrito of the olive oil, onions, garlic and red, orange and green peppers are just sautéed Paleo. You can also try ground beef, tomatoes, sliced potatoes and spices to give a different but great taste sensation.

For a dessert, you can bake some apples slices with cinnamon and walnuts.

**Snacks**

The best snacks to eat early in the afternoon are fresh fruits such as bananas, apples strawberries and blueberries. You can also try guacamole together with raw broccoli plus carrots, peanuts, almonds, cashew, or even a homemade jerky.

All dairy products such as yogurt, milk and cheese are excluded in this died. Coffee, legumes and alcohol are also not allowed in your daily intake.

The Paleo diet is simple and only requires you to eat healthy and natural food. This diet has no calorie counting therefore ideal for those who want lose weight. It does not require you to purchase any expensive pre- packaged food, all you need to carefully plan your meals and then prepare them. Other benefits of Paleo diet includes a smoother, healthier skin, increased energy and a deeper and much more restful sleep. Remember to consult with your doctor for more advice.

# CHAPTER 8- PALEO DIET- COMMON MISTAKES TO AVOID

What follows are some of the most common mistakes while on the Paleo diet that people are making every single day and the idea behind informing you of these mistakes is to help stop you from making the exact same ones yourself and undoing all of the good work that you have already put into your diet regime. There is no doubt that this particular diet can have some amazing results when it is done correctly, so read on in order to find out more about what you should not do.

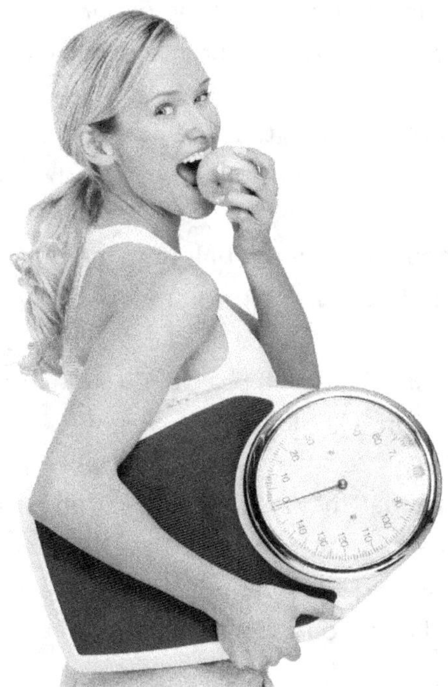

First, people will often try to completely eliminate fat from their diet as they believe that it is evil and will result in them putting on weight rather than losing it. The truth of the matter is that you need some of it in your diet as it makes you feel more full and helps to absorb various nutrients and minerals in your food, so include some without going crazy and you will benefit from doing so.

Another mistake is that they try to make everything about the Paleo diet and this will then put undue pressure on their body as we all naturally crave different things as some kind of treat every now and then.

The problem is that so many people go from one extreme to the other when in actual fact you can have that little treat at different times as long as it does not become a mainstay in your diet because the main focus of this type of diet has to be on eating more natural meat and vegetables for the majority of your food with little tit-bits thrown in to keep your interest alive.

People are also guilty of thinking that they can eat as many nuts as they like because surely nuts have to be part of the Paleo diet?

In actual fact, you should look at limiting the amount of nuts you eat because they do not actually help you to lose any weight, so if you are having them as a snack, then always make sure that they are small portions rather than a big bag or you will undo the hard work you have already put in to lose some weight.

Finally, people believe that they need to eat less in order to lose weight on this diet because they believe that the idea is that in the Paleolithic era food was scarce, which then leads to binges rather than controlled meals on a regular basis.

This is the wrong way to do things because you need to eat small meals on a regular basis and make sure that you get enough fats and protein in order to give your body the fuel it needs to actually work. Binging in your diet will only result in your metabolism going haywire and losing weight will become extremely difficult as a result so small meals on a regular basis is undoubtedly the way forward.

People, therefore, make these common mistakes while on the Paleo diet and you can see that in order to avoid making them it simply involves you taking that little bit more care and fully understanding what the diet involves before you even start it. By taking your time you will not only manage to lose weight, but will also be healthier as well and benefit from it not only now, but in the long- term as well

# CHAPTER 9- HOW TO SHOP FOR FOOD?

Shopping for food on the Paleo diet doesn't have to be difficult. If you're on a budget then there is a simple plan you can follow to get the healthiest food for your money. First, prioritize animal protein, and then move on to vegetables followed by fruits and lastly fats.

Animal protein is where you want to spend the bulk of your budget. Always go for organic grass-fed or pasteurized meat. Buy it fresh and buy what is available. If you can't find organic grass fed lamb but you see organic beef, then buy the beef and change your dinner recipe for that night. If you see organic chicken on special, then buy a bunch of them and eat chicken all week, or freeze some of them.

If your budget is too tight to afford the best quality, try to stick to meat from ruminants (beef, lamb, venison, goat, buffalo etc). These animals feed on their natural diet for at least a portion of their lives. Their meat also has a better ratio of Omega-6 to Omega-3 than meat like pork or chicken.

It's best to buy the leanest cuts and trim the fat from them. Many of the unhealthy things like environmental toxins, hormones and antibiotics reside in the fat, so it should be trimmed or drained before consumption.

Always eat non-organic chicken without the skin for the same reasons. It's best to avoid pork altogether if you can't buy organic.

The next source of animal protein is fish. Since this will only last for a day at home, don't overspend here. Buy enough for one meal unless you are planning to freeze it. Wild-caught fish is good but pricey. You can buy less expensive fish that is often just as good like cod or scallops. Look at frozen fish as well; these are often a good substitute to the pricey stuff.

The final source for animal protein is eggs. There is only one rule here; buy organic. They are more expensive than "cage free" eggs but even so, they are still one of your cheapest sources of high quality protein.

Once you have your animal protein sorted, it's time to look at fruit and vegetables. It is not always best to buy organic. It's better to spend less on fruits and vegetables and more on better quality meat. A little pesticide on your produce is tolerable if it means you get high quality protein from meat, fish and eggs.

As a general rule, always buy in season and buy what's on special. Get your vegetables sorted before you purchase fruit. You can do without fruit if necessary but you need to eat your veggies. Buy dark, leafy vegetables, as they are more nutrient-rich. Stay away from vegetables like lettuce, celery and cucumbers, as they don't have much nutrition. To save money you can also purchase frozen vegetables.

The next stop is fats. Dietary fat can be expensive so don't go crazy on things like nuts and seeds. Coconut products are good, inexpensive source of fats, especially coconut milk. In addition, avocados are a good source of fat and are available all year round. Olives preserved in salt and water is also a good choice. These are the staples for fats so go for them first. If you still have some room in your budget, you can buy nuts and seeds last.

When your budget allows, you can go for higher priced items like cold-pressed extra-virgin olive oil, unrefined coconut oil and organic pastured butter. These are all good sources of fat and they can last for months.

The last thing you may want to consider is stocking up on herbs and spices. They can be expensive but, adding a little to your spice rack each week will make eating chicken five nights a week much more interesting.

# CHAPTER 10- HOW TO EXERCISE WHILE ON THE PALEO DIET

Combating fat can be done by anyone irrespective of age if you follow a strict Paleo diet. It does matter if you are a man or a woman. You can simply burn off all the fat that made you look chubby in as little as 3 workouts everyday if you can eat right. You don't even need to visit the gym. Most diet programs prevent you from eating what you want. They restrict your calorie intake that can lead to destruction of your metabolism.

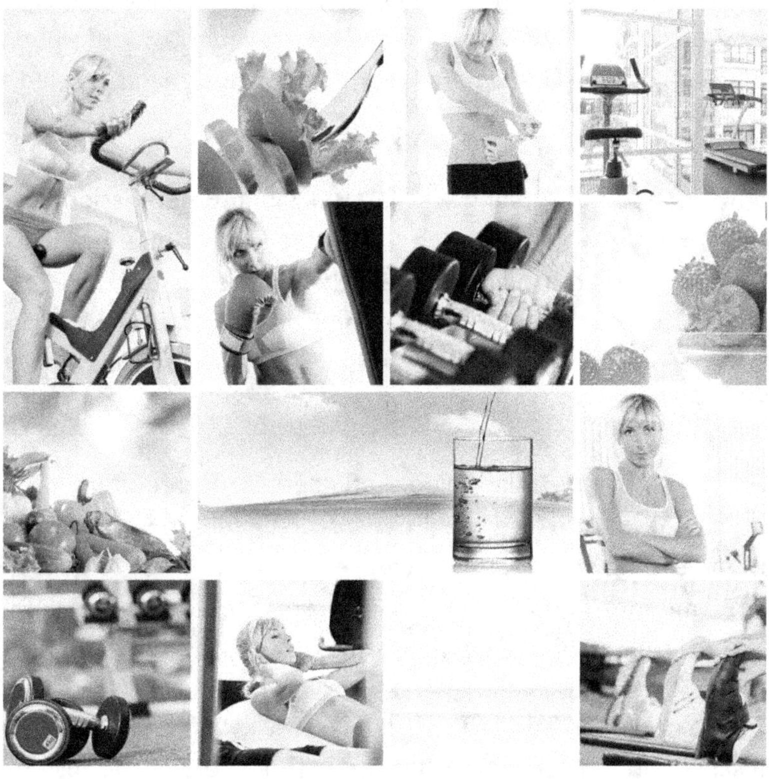

However Paleo diet allows your body to derive enough nutrition from food to help you benefit from a workout and also keeps you going.

If you think that Paleo diet is only for skinny guys and cannot put on weight or cannot build that poster perfect body that you have always dreamed of then you are not right. All that was said in the magazines, popular muscle building shows by renowned body builders, don't seem to be working.

All the books that I was reading made me feel that I could never be fit and will always be the skinny guy I was born. Despite what I did, weight gain was a far cry leave alone muscle building. Despite being taunted by my hunky friends I persevered. I spent a lot of money on health supplements month after month and slogged at the gym.

I almost had given up and was fast sinking into depression when one of my hunky and taunting roommates let me in on the Paleo diet and a workout plan. The rest they say is history. It takes a while to understand the regimen and one read will not suffice. However in essence it suggests that proper eating combined with light workout can really make a difference.

With a healthy diet like Paleo diet, there is no requirement for intense workout to lose weight as the diet itself does most of the job in keeping you healthy. However if you do seek to gain the extra amount of fitness, you need to consider working out with a personal trainer who understands the diet you are on.

Most people who intend to workout heavily want to pile on the muscle rapidly. That cannot happen with Paleo diet because it is natural and does not cause artificial building of muscle. However when combined with a fitness workout plan that aims to improve your heart, the lungs and overall muscle tone the Paleo diet is very useful.

**Workout Your Heart And Lungs**

Cardio exercises that aim to improve the function of the heart are most effective with Paleo diet. This will not just help you reduce weight but also make it stronger. You can take up simple exercises like the jogging and running. Running is best suited for staying naturally fit as it helps workout the entire body. The heart is worked effectively because heart rate is made to vary through the workout session. The impact of the workout on the entire body is high as it helps in connective tissue building and strengthening of bones. Despite all the modern workout machines we have at our disposal, it is ideal for burning calories.

Cycling is another activity I would suggest for the heart. You can burn about 500 calories in less than an hour through cycling. It also helps build muscle in both lower and upper body. Besides, just like running the heart benefits are immense.

Regular swimming when on Paleo diet is very beneficial. Swimming helps improve blood circulation and also improves lung capacity. Swimming also helps in building of the muscles and joints of the arms and the legs.

Because the Paleo diet is not meant to help you pump muscle, solely relying on it for body building is not beneficial. However the idea of body building itself goes against the principles of Paleo Diet. Diet, as taken by our ancestors was meant to keep them fit and strong not make huge. Hence the diet cannot give you the body if you desire to beef up. However it is possible for you to indulge in light workout sessions which will help you gain an even muscle tone but activities like bench press cannot be sustained on simple Paleo diet.

*Paleo Diet Plan*

Apart from working out your heart and lungs you can also consider repetitive workouts of push-ups, light weight lifting and activities like kick boxing. Martial arts are also a good workout plan when on Paleo diet. However having a personal trainer to guide you through

A regular massage is really beneficial when on Paleo diet. A massage can lead to a high state of relaxation which will lower defenses of the mind. Hence it is possible that you may find yourself crying on narrating a tragedy. Let your emotions pour out. By the end of it, with your mind relaxed you will feel light and relieved. Avoid the urge to have alcohol or any other intoxicant. This will defeat the whole purpose. It is good to drink water after a massage. Water will help complement the massage. A massage leads to surfacing of toxins from your tissues. To facilitate their exit, water is needed.

With food in the stomach, your body metabolism cannot relax and this could render the massage ineffective. Hence it is advisable to not eat anything 45 minutes prior to the massage. The objective of a massage is to relax the body and mind. There should be no distractions that can disturb your state. Try and drop disturbing thoughts about work and life. If music soothes you then you can a light instrumental playing in the back ground. Also chose a fragrance of your choice for aroma therapy.

# CHAPTER 11-HEALTHY PALEO RECIPES

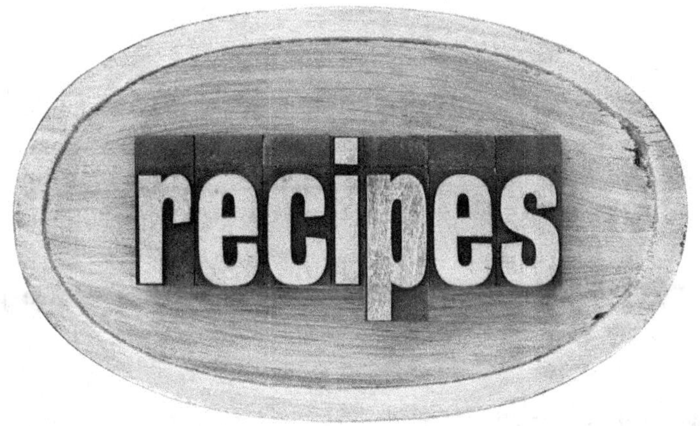

**Paleo Pancake**

6 eggs

1 can coconut milk

2 Teaspoons vanilla

1/2 Tablespoon baking soda

1 Tablespoon honey

2 Teaspoons cinnamon

3/4 Cup coconut flour

Instructions:

Preparing this pancake is simple. This is healthy and does not require much time. All you have to do is beat the eggs until they're frothy and mix the remaining ingredients together. Set the heat to medium and cook on the girdle. When you pour the batter, try to keep the cakes small.

**Paleo Chips**

1 large, ripe eggplant
2 Eggs
2 cups

Instructions:

Shred the egg plant in a food processor. Mix it with egg and cheese. Bake (on both sides) the mixture at 450 degrees F in a pre-heated oven for 10 minutes. Loosen and flip the circles. Remove from oven and cut rounds into triangles with a pizza cutter. Allow it cool before being served.

**Broccoli and Pine-Nut Soup**

1 onion, diced
1tbs oil
3 cups broccoli
3 cups chicken or vegetable stock
¼ cup pine-nuts

Instructions:

Start by frying the onion in a large pan with oil on medium heat until slightly browned. After the onion has been moderately browned, add the broccoli and the stock. Let the mixture simmer for 10-15 minutes or until broccoli has softened. Set it aside and let it cool down for a short time. Take your broccoli and stock mixture and place it in a food processor or use an electric blender. Process or blend until you have created a smooth texture. Remember to heat your soup before serving it to your guests or family.

**Paleo Apple Recipe**

*Andryan Coombs*
2 large apples
2 cups strawberries
1 tsp cinnamon
¼ cup purified water

Instructions:

Clean, core and dice apples. Add diced apples and strawberries in a blender and add a ¼ cup of purified water and cinnamon and process about 30 seconds or until smooth. Pour mixture on a teflex sheet (a Teflon-coated sheet commonly used to dehydrate delicate foods) and place in a plastic dehydrator. Dehydrate for 6-8 hours, remove teflex and flip fruit. Continue drying another 4-6 hours or until desired consistency is achieved. Use a pizza cutter to slice into snack-size pieces.

**Italian-Style Roast Beef**

4-pound bottom round roast
2 large onions, sliced
3 cloves garlic, chopped
1 tablespoon garlic powder, plus more to taste
1 tablespoon oregano, plus more to taste
2 cups fresh baby carrots

Instructions:

In Dutch oven, sear sides of roast over high heat until well browned. Brown in a few Tbs. of oil in the Dutch oven on medium high heat, on all sides. Remove from pan and set aside. Lower heat to medium and add onion and garlic, cooking about 3 minutes until softened. Season meat with garlic powder and oregano and return to pan. Add one cup cold water to pan.

Cover and cook on medium-low heat for about 3 1/2 hours. Add more water as needed to create a rich au jus. After the second hour, arrange baby carrots around the meat, seasoning with garlic powder and oregano to taste. When meat is tender, remove from meat, carrots and onions from pan. Put meat on a carving board and slice; place carrots in serving bowl with cooked onion.

## Kale Chips Recipe

2 handfuls kale leaves
1 teaspoon cayenne pepper
Cooking spray
Sea salt

Instructions:

Preheat oven to 350°F. Arrange kale on a non stick baking sheet. Very lightly coat kale with cooking spray and a bit of sea salt. Sprinkle cayenne pepper on top of the kale and bake for 10 minutes or until crispy.

## Paleo Egg Breakfast

Two eggs
5 to 7 slices of bacon
One handful of frozen spinach

Instructions:

Boil the eggs. I like to boil mine for about 6 minutes and then immediately put them under cold water. Put the bacon slices in a frying pan. You won't need grease, the bacon is greasy enough. The frozen spinach (or fresh if you have that available) could be unfreezes in the microwave for 2 to 3 minutes. Add some salt on top of the eggs and you are good to go.

**Roasted Acorn Squash Recipe**

2 acorn/pepper squash;
3 tbsp clarified butter, tallow or coconut oil;
2 onions, thinly sliced;
3 cloves garlic, minced;
1 tsp ground coriander seed;
½ tsp nutmeg;
Sea salt and freshly ground black pepper to taste;

Instructions:

Preheat your oven to 375 F. Cut each squash in half, but leave the seeds in. Place cut end up on a baking sheet and roast them for about 50 minutes to an hour, long enough so that the flesh is fork tender. Remove once cooked and let cool for several minutes. Meanwhile, in a medium skillet over a medium heat, sauté the onions in the cooking fat. Cook for close to 10 minutes, until the onions are translucent and begin to be golden brown. Add the garlic to the skillet, followed by the coriander, nutmeg, salt and pepper. Continue to cook for about 2 minutes. Remove the seeds from the squash and discard. Spoon out the tender flesh and discard the skin. Roughly mash up the squash and add it to the skillet. Mix well. Only leave on heat long enough to blend flavors.

**Boiled Fish**

Fish filets (1-2 per serving)

Salt
Pepper
Garlic salt

*Paleo Diet Plan*
Lime or lemon
Fresh or frozen broccoli

Instructions:

First you want to find fish filets with white flesh, they should be pretty firm and have no strong fishy smell. The best way is to ask in your grocery store which day they get fish delivery and time your shopping accordingly. Pre-heat the oven to 350 degrees F (175 degrees C). While the oven is heated you can prepare the fish by putting it in a greased broiling pan and squeeze the lime over it. Add some salt, pepper and maybe a touch of garlic salt to it.

The broiling time can vary quite a bit depending on how big the filets are. If we are using fresh filets u broil them about 10 to 12 minutes. The easiest way to tell if the fish is done is to use a fork. When it flakes easily it is ready to be served. It takes about 4-5 minutes in the microwave oven to unfreeze them. Add some light sea salt to it and your ready to go!

**Cinnamon Chicken Recipe**

1 3lbs chicken, cut into 8 pieces (breasts, drumsticks, thighs and wings);

½ tsp sea salt;
½ tsp black pepper;
2/3 tsp cinnamon;
2 cloves garlic, minced;
½ tsp paprika;
1 onion, sliced;
1 cup water or chicken stock;

Instructions:

*Andryan Coombs*

Preheat your oven to 400 F. In a small bowl, combine the salt, pepper, garlic and cinnamon. Rub the chicken pieces with this mixture and allow it to sit for about 30 minutes at room temperature. Place the chicken pieces in a large roasting pan, sprinkle the meat all over with the paprika and add the onion slices to the pan. Cook for 35 minutes and then reduce the heat to 350 F. Stir in a cup of water to the roasting pan and continue cooking for another 50 minutes. Serve and use the juices from the pan as a sauce.

**Carob Treat**

1 cup toasted unsweetened carob
1 ½ cups pecan meal
½ cup or less coconut oil

Instructions:

In a large bowl, mix all ingredients together. Spread in a baking tin lined with parchment paper.

**Shrimp Ceviche**

1 lb. shrimp, peeled & deveined
4 limes
1 small shallot, diced
1 medium tomato, diced
1 jalapeno, seeded and minced
1/4 cup olive oil
1 tsp. kosher salt
1/2 tsp. fresh ground black pepper
1/4 cup fresh cilantro leaves, diced
1 avocado

Instructions:

Bring a pot of water to boil and cook shrimp for about 3 minutes, until just cooked. Cooked shrimp ready for the lime juice. Drain, cool, de-tail, and roughly chop shrimp.

Squeeze limes into a medium bowl. Add shrimp, shallot, tomato, jalapeno, olive oil, salt, and pepper to lime juice and combine well. Cover and let marinate in fridge for a minimum of one hour (can chill up to six). Stir cilantro into chilled mixture. Serve ceviche with a slotted spoon and top with 1/4 sliced avocado.

# CONCLUSION

As we conclude this guide we must remember that the Paleo diet is a consumption plan designed to replicate the nutritional habits of humans' hunter-gatherer ancestors. It is based on the principle that human beings might attain better health and optimal weight by avoiding diets high in carbohydrates and sugar and instead eating a lot of lean meats, fish, fruits and vegetables. Below are 6 tips to help you start the Paleo diet today:

**Awareness**

You get a pretty excellent idea of what the Paleo diet is all about by researching on the internet, books, journals or joining Paleo groups in the different social networking sites such as Facebook, twitter and meetuip.com. You should know which foods the Paleo diet avoids also.

Advocates of the Paleo diet believe that there is a direct association between the increasing prevalence of several chronic diseases, like obesity, diabetes as well as heart disease, with the increasing intake of carbohydrates and sugar. Advocates recommend eating a diet like that of our hunter-gatherer ancestors where foods like sugar, bread, pasta, cereals, dairy products, trans fats and fatty meats were not available as the only way to attain better health.

Moreover, advocates recommend us to keep away from starchy vegetables like corn and potatoes, legumes, peanuts, beans, and every type of fruit juices and sodas.

**Identify the Best Paleo Diet Foods**

*Paleo Diet Plan*

A Paleo diet is rich in protein, a nutrient which enhances satiety and increases weight loss better compared to processed carbohydrates. The best Paleo diet foods should incorporate chicken, fish, shellfish, avocados, eggs, nuts, berries, turnips and carrots.

**Include Paleo Diet in Your Everyday Plan**

Arrange how you'll include the Paleo diet in your everyday plan. Foods high in carbohydrate, whole grains foods are easily accessible in fast-food cafe and vending machines, however Paleo diet foods are difficult to get. Less Paleo foods are kept in a pantry. Get into the pantry and remove all processed food, such as rice, beans, bread, sugar, cereals, pasta, candy, sodas, cake mixes and potato chips that is kept there. Donate unopened and usable products to local food pantry or either throws it all away or feasts on it for some days to eliminate it. An effective start of the Paleo diet implies scheduling the foods you'll take for breakfast, lunch as well as dinner. In this way, you'll not be prone to reaching for processed foods once hungry.

**Get Ready For the Effects of Radically Reducing Carbohydrate Intake**

People taking a diet rich in carbohydrates might experience a range of consequences when commencing a Paleo diet. It can result to dizziness, tiredness and constipation. Moreover, a Paleo diet might stimulate ketosis, a condition which leads to rapid breakdown of body fat. This might be particularly risky for expectant women and individuals suffering from diabetes.

**Gradual Transition**

Slowly shun your processed food intake patterns and substitute them with Paleo diet foods. You can take up even a month. A best way to include this is to avoid purchasing any processed foods once you go to the market.

**Detox**

A best way to start a Paleo diet is to detox your body first. You can simply cleanse your body by taking just water together with lemon juice, cayenne pepper and maple syrup for a period of between 1-7 days.

Well that brings us to the end of this beginners guide to the Paleo diet, Go out and take charge of your life and your diet

# ABOUT THE AUTHOR

Andryan Coombs was always a little overweight and she was always trying to find the perfect diet that would give the long terms effects of weight loss and improved health and wellness. That is how she found the Paleo diet. It was not a fasting diet and it was filled with nutritious meal options.

As a nutritionist in training she knew that this would have some benefits so she tried and proved found it to be extremely beneficial. That is what she promotes in her books. It is not about starving but about modifying the diet and including exercise to make the weight loss effective.